I0791974

Table of Contents

What Is DMSO?

DMSO (Dimethyl Sulfoxide) is derived from dimethyl sulfide, a by-product in the manufacturing of paper products from Pine trees. It is widely used to replace sulfur in the human body. It is also used as a pain remedy. DMSO loves to eat up the free radicals in your body that cause inflammation. Rather than masking the pain, DMSO actually reduces inflammation and prevents free radical damage.

DMSO's uses are seemingly endless in the area of pain management. People who have been using the solvent are also reporting other health improvements that they were not expecting. DMSO has been used successfully in conjunction with the following diagnosis:

Arthritis

Immune System Disorders like MS and Lupus

Atherosclerosis (narrowing of arteries)

Cataracts, Eye Inflammation, Retinol Disease, Macular Degeneration

Herpes and Shingles

Interstitial cystitis (painful bladder condition)

FDA approved use

Scleroderma (hardening of the skin)

Wound Care

Psoriasis, Eczema and other skin disorders

Dementia and Alzheimer's

Our soil has been depleted of life-giving sulfur. This has caused us to be deficient. Sulfur can be found in almost every cell and is very important to maintain good health. Sulfur is the third most abundant mineral element found in our bodies. Low sulfur levels in the body have been linked to many health issues including low levels of Glutathione. Glutathione has protective role against oxidative and free radical damage and its potential to enhance the immune function.

Insulin disorders, inflammation, immune system disorders and weak joints are just a few of the areas that DMSO can help. As a supplement, sulfur is available in two forms: dimethyl sulfoxide (DMSO) and methylsulfonylmethane (MSM). DMSO is the liquid form and MSM comes in a crystal form or powder. Used together you can have a powerful antioxidant that can help with free radical damage and inflammation.

MSM for joint pain

If you decide to purchase DMSO you will want to get 99.99% Pure Pharmaceutical Grade DMSO in a glass bottle or jar. In that form you will want to dilute it with distilled water. Veterinarians also use DMSO to help with pain management. Often used with horses and other animals it is most likely industrial grade and should not be used by humans.

Always get DMSO in a glass bottle

Always store DMSO in glass

How Do I Use DMSO?

DMSO comes in a liquid form. It can be taken internally with an IV or orally and may also be used topically. You will find it for sale in its pure liquid form or with another substance like Aloe Vera. If you purchase it in its pure liquid form you will want to dilute it. Depending on what you are using it for, many will add essential oils, distilled water or Aloe Vera.

You can purchase DMSO at local health food stores and on Amazon. I personally have it in 2 forms. There is a pure liquid form in a glass bottle. It can be taken orally or topically that can be diluted with distilled water or other substances. Then I have a jar that is a 70/30 dilution with Aloe Vera that can go on topically. You can test your liquid DMSO for purity when it arrives. Pure DMSO will crystalize below 66F. Just put your bottle in the refrigerator over night and you will see crystals form. To warm it up just run the bottle under warm tap water.

DMSO can be irritating to the skin. You will not want to put it on at full strength as it can cause redness and itching. Even diluted you will have an itching sensation for about 15 minutes after application. Repeated use can also dry the skin. This is a small price to pay for a natural supplement that has so many benefits. Prescriptions and over the counter pain medications that are wreaking havoc on our bodies.

DMSO is a carrier compound. DMSO has the ability to rapidly penetrate the skin. This also means that it opens a gateway for other substances to enter the body through the skin. Because it is a carrier, you must use DMSO on clean skin and not have it come in contact with any other substances such as your clothes or furniture. The DMSO will carry whatever it touches right through your skin. That includes dirt and chemicals that you do not want inside your body. Once it is in your system it attaches itself to the free radicals and eliminates them.

DMSO has the ability to break through the blood-brain barrier. It is being studied in patients with Alzheimer's and dementia. This property has allowed for its use in drug therapies. DMSO is water-soluble. It can carry the drugs to areas that it can not normally be reached without doing any damage.

Side Effects of DMSO

DMSO can have a couple of minor side effects that can be annoying but are manageable.

DMSO Can Cause You to Smell

Many people report that their breath and body odor will start to smell like garlic or oysters. From my research, holistic health professionals, state that it is their opinion that this happens when you have more toxins. Others report that it only happens when you take it internally. Either way, you can manage the odors with peppermint gum and essential oils.

I have no idea if it is the toxins, but it is something that can be an issue for a few days after your last application or dose. The problem with it is that you can not smell it on yourself, so you will need to have a friend or a spouse keep an eye on it for you.

DMSO Is Itchy

When I used it on my back it was a struggle. Not only did I have to lay on my stomach to make sure nothing was touching the DMSO, like clothing or bedding, it also made me itch like crazy. Some say that this goes away in time. I was using a 70/30 ratio with Aloe Vera which did not dry quickly and is pretty strong. At a 50/50 ratio of DMSO and distilled water, it dried faster so it made it more manageable.

Supplement with Minerals

Many holistic health practitioners recommend that you supplement with magnesium or Trace Minerals when using DMSO. Many people will mix DMSO with Magnesium oil which is also anti-inflammatory. When starting with DMSO it is important to start slow and allow your body to adjust.

11 Great Ways to Use DMSO

MSM and DSMO used together are a powerful antioxidant and pain reliever.

Essential oils used with DMSO go deeper into your cells and can penetrate the blood brain barrier.

Detox your liver with Castor Oil and DMSO.

20% DMSO and 80% distilled water eyedrops can improve many eye diseases such as cataracts.

Castor Oil in the eyes before bed can also help to soften cataracts.

DMSO contains oxygen so it is antimicrobial, anti-viral and anti-fungal. You can use it for toe fungus, athletes foot, acne and other skin conditions.

DMSO on your scalp may help regenerate hair growth in some people.

Eliminate bruising and scars. I noticed immediate results on my newer scars. On my older scars it took about 6 weeks . Apply your 70/30 solution 2-3 times per day for best results.

A teaspoon of DMSO with orange juice taken daily can improve your overall health.

I have seen many testimonials from people who have suffered from strokes who have taken DMSO internally and REVERSED the damage if done soon enough.

Use a 20% solution of DMSO in conjunction with Vitamin C in your skin care regimen for younger looking skin and wrinkles.

A 50/50 solution of DMSO and distilled water around the temples and base of the neck has been reported to stop migraines if used at the onset.

What are the Different DMSO Uses?

A liquid chemical solvent known as dimethyl sulfoxide or DMSO may be a modern day cure-all or a potentially hazardous example of quack medicine. Derived from wood pulp, DMSO was first tested as a possible pharmaceutical drug in the early 1960s. Preliminary test results showed that DMSO had the ability to penetrate organic membranes such as skin tissue, blood vessels and human organs. Because these membranes could be penetrated by DMSO without damage, some researchers believed the chemical compound could be used as a more effective drug delivery system, since pain-killing medicines such as morphine sulfate could be mixed with DMSO and applied to the patient's skin. Other medications could also be piggybacked with DMSO, such as anti-inflammatory or cancer-fighting drugs.

DMSO may be effective in treating the pain and swelling associated with arthritis.

DMSO may be effective in treating the pain and swelling associated with arthritis.

DMSO uses include topical skin treatments, minor muscular ailments and anti-viral applications. Skin conditions such as acne, psoriasis, and dermatitis could be treated with regular applications of DMSO. Minor burns and skin rashes are also said to be treatable with DMSO. DMSO has antioxidant properties and is considered a free radical scavenger, which means it has the ability to penetrate cell walls and flood them with oxygen. This action creates a hostile environment for viruses, since they depend on the cells for duplication. Topical skin conditions also benefit from the increase in oxygenation and the elimination of damaging free radicals.

The Federal Food and Drug Administration has only approved the use of DMSO for interstitial cystitis, a condition characterized by bladder inflammation.

The Federal Food and Drug Administration has only approved the use of DMSO for interstitial cystitis, a condition characterized by bladder inflammation.

Other DMSO uses are more controversial, but also promising, according to many DMSO proponents. Some claim that DMSO has a positive effect on such painful and debilitating conditions such as scleroderma and arthritis. Because DMSO can penetrate joint tissue and destroy free radicals, it may relieve much of the swelling and pain associated with arthritis. Some studies suggest that arthritis patients who were administered DMSO demonstrated a greater range of motion and significantly less joint pain following treatment. DMSO can also soften collagen, a natural substance which gives skin its elastic qualities. Some scleroderma patients reported shrinking of inflamed tissue after receiving several applications of DMSO. However, the Federal Food and Drug Administration (FDA) has only approved the use of DMSO for one condition, interstitial cystitis.

DMSO may be helpful in treating pain associated with minor burns.

DMSO may be helpful in treating pain associated with minor burns.

Some DMSO uses are still a source of controversy for proponents and critics alike. DMSO has been used for decades as a liniment for horses, and many human athletes have also been treated with DMSO after suffering muscle cramps or sprained joints. During the 1970s and early 1980s, many people illicitly purchased bottles of DMSO as an alternative cure-all for conditions ranging from cuts and scrapes to advanced forms of cancer. Because industrial grade DMSO was not legally approved for non-prescription human use, many DMSO marketers were investigated and/or prosecuted. Medicinal-grade DMSO can still be obtained from alternative health stores and other online sources. A derivative of DMSO called Methyl Sulfonyl Methane (MSM) is also marketed as a dietary supplement, with its own laundry list of uses and benefits. Because DMSO and MSM are marketed primarily as dietary supplements and not medications, they are not subject to the same scrutiny and regulation of prescription or over-the-counter medicines. It is important for consumers to research a product such as DMSO thoroughly before deciding whether or not to use it for health purposes.

What other things can DMSO be used for?

young woman with red hair holding elbow in pain, joint pain DMSO can help with a number of different issues and conditions. This includes all of the following:

Inflammatory diseases.

Joint pain relief

Cancer side-effects (pain)

Gastrointestinal disorders

Headaches and migraines

Fibromyalgia

Shingles

Psoriasis

Candida

Eczema

Tendonitis

Arthritis

Interstitial cystitis

Autoimmune disorders

Hemorrhoid

Muscle spasms

And more!

DMSO and Flap Perfusion in Plastic Surgery

In 1968, McFarlane et al2 reported on the use of DMSO to prevent necrosis in experimental pedicle flaps; numerous studies that followed confirmed this discovery.3–6 The mechanism of action is not fully understood, but DMSO is known to stimulate histamine release,7,8 and histamine release triggers vasodilation.

Both topical and intravenous DMSO solutions have been studied in animal models of pedicle, island, and cutaneous flaps. One study of abdominal island flaps in rats compared control animals that received saline injections with rats injected with intraperitoneal DMSO. Flaps in the treatment group showed significantly increased blood perfusion by postoperative day 3 as measured by laser Doppler velocimetry and perfusion fluorometry.4

In another controlled rat study, 9 × 4-cm pedicle flaps were elevated on the abdomen. The epigastric vein was occluded with a clamp for 8 hours before the clamp was removed and the flap resutured to its bed.9 Two groups of animals received intraperitoneal saline. Three groups received intraperitoneal DMSO at different timepoints: (1) at reperfusion only; (2) at reperfusion and then every day for 5 days; or (3) before surgery, at reperfusion, and for 5 days after surgery. The area of flap survival was measured with a sonic digitizer. When administered as a single dose at reperfusion, DMSO did not increase flap survival compared with controls receiving saline. However, both groups receiving DMSO at reperfusion and for 5 postoperative days had a significantly greater percentage of flap survival area: 78% to 86% for DMSO versus 32% to 34% for saline (P < 0.01).

The survival of skin flaps with topically applied DMSO was also investigated. In this model, 10 × 2.5-cm flaps were elevated and then resutured on the backs of rabbits.6 Four groups were compared: (1) those treated with saline; (2) those treated with 8% hydrogen peroxide (H2O2); (3) those treated with 50% DMSO; and (4) those treated with 50% DMSO + 8% H2O2. DMSO with H2O2 was studied because H2O2 stimulates the release of oxygen when applied to tissues, and DMSO penetrates cell membranes; so, theoretically, DMSO could deliver hydrogen peroxide throughout the flap. Treatments were topically administered 3 times daily for 7 days, beginning immediately after surgery. Transcutaneous oxygen tension (PtcO2) in the flaps was measured 72 hours after surgery, and the percentage of surviving skin area was measured by planimetry 7 days after flap elevation.

There were no significant differences in area of flap survival for the groups that received saline (71% survival), 8% H2O2 (72% survival), or 50% DMSO (76% survival). However, flaps that received the combination of DMSO + H2O2 had a significantly larger area of survival (92%). The mean PtcO2 value also was significantly different for the DMSO + H2O2 group (95% versus 74% for the other 3 groups).

Reported clinical studies of DMSO and flap survival have thus far been limited to mastectomy patients. Rand-Luby et al10 performed a randomized, prospective study of skin flap viability in patients undergoing mastectomy and inguinal lymphadenectomy. Twenty-four patients treated with 60% DMSO topically applied to their flaps every 4 hours for 10 days after surgery were compared with 27 patients who had surgery alone. The maximum area of flap ischemia was traced by a masked observer and measured by cut and weigh technique. The mean area of ischemia for the DMSO-treated group was 16.3 U versus 44.9 U for the controls (P = 0.01).

Tissue expansion in patients undergoing immediate breast reconstruction following modified radical mastectomy was studied by Raposio and Santi11 to determine whether DMSO could reduce expander pressure and length of treatment. One group of 20 patients underwent standard tissue expansion, and in another group of 20 patients, 60% DMSO-soaked surgical sponges were left on the skin overlying the expander for 30 minutes prior to expansion. A statistically significant difference in the number of weekly expander filling sessions was found, with a mean of 6 sessions for the untreated group and a mean of 4 sessions for the DMSO-treated group. In addition, there was a significant difference in the average inflated volume per session; the untreated group had an average of 90 mL added to their expanders per session, compared with the DMSO-treated group who had an average of 120 mL added to their expanders per session. The ability to complete tissue expansion more quickly following mastectomy can be considered a real benefit for these patients.

Vinnik[5] has reported that he achieves maximal tissue expansion in minutes by applying topical DMSO, which permits immediate placement of large permanent implants after mastectomy. He also uses topical DMSO to maximize the area of skin resection in patients undergoing abdominoplasty, thereby maintaining good flap perfusion.

We have observed skin perfusion improvement with topical application of DMSO following abdominoplasty and face lift procedures. Figure 1 demonstrates the immediate and obvious impact of DMSO on skin perfusion in a woman undergoing abdominoplasty. We would like to emphasize, however, that we do not recommend using DMSO as a way to increase the area of resection during surgery. DMSO should be used to increase perfusion. Resection should always be kept within safe margins.

A, DMSO 99% was applied to the right side immediately after abdominoplasty closure. B, Same patient 12 minutes later. Skin perfusion on the right is obviously increased. The 2 photos were not taken from the exact same angle, but the effects of DMSO are evident.

Open in new tabDownload slide

A, DMSO 99% was applied to the right side immediately after abdominoplasty closure. B, Same patient 12 minutes later. Skin perfusion on the right is obviously increased. The 2 photos were not taken from the exact same angle, but the effects of DMSO are evident.

A, DMSO 99% was applied to the right side immediately after abdominoplasty closure. B,

Same patient 12 minutes later. Skin perfusion on the right is obviously increased. The 2 photos were not taken from the exact same angle, but the effects of DMSO are evident.

A, DMSO 99% was applied to the right side immediately after abdominoplasty closure. B, Same patient 12 minutes later. Skin perfusion on the right is obviously increased. The 2 photos were not taken from the exact same angle, but the effects of DMSO are evident.

It seems reasonable to try DMSO when other more traditional methods of improving circulation, such as releasing tension, relieving kinks from pedicles, or decreasing pressure, have failed. If an area shows signs of ischemia or appears to have inadequate perfusion, application of topical DMSO, every 4 to 6 hours until blood flow improves, should be beneficial. The product is inexpensive and easy for patients to use at home. Although DMSO probably cannot repair areas of necrosis, it may prevent loss of circulation in ischemic tissues or decrease the size of a possibly necrotic area.

Experimental studies have found DMSO to be effective in tissue ischemia related to either arterial or venous obstruction. Consequently, the cause of ischemia should not be a consideration when contemplating DMSO treatment.

Concentrations of topically applied DMSO in the flap studies cited vary from 50% and 60% to our use of 99%. The literature review indicates that the ability of DMSO to cross all membranes varies according to DMSO strength. The most effective DMSO strength for penetrating skin is a solution between 70% and 90%.12,13 For reasons unknown, concentrations higher than 90% are less effective. Our choice of DMSO concentration will be less than 90% in the future. Much lower concentrations of DMSO—in the range of 1% to 8%—are sufficient for crossing membranes other than skin.

The 60% DMSO concentration used in the context of tissue expansion following mastectomy10,11 may have been chosen because lower concentrations can minimize skin reactions, which could be especially important when the skin above an expander is soaked in DMSO for 30 minutes. (Even a 60% DMSO concentration produced impressive results in these studies.) In our experience, topical use of DMSO has been limited to a few days at most, and no skin irritation has been seen. Any erythema or wheal that did occur should disappear soon after DMSO treatments are stopped.

Other Possible DMSO Applications in Plastic Surgery

Keloids

Biopsies of keloids have shown histologic improvement after DMSO treatment.14 Thus, DMSO may be effective for this difficult problem.

Pain relief

Several animal studies have explored the analgesic action of DMSO,13,15,16 which seems to block peripheral nerve C fibers.17 One study found that DMSO was not only as effective as morphine for pain relief, but that its effect persisted several hours longer than that of morphine.18 DMSO also has been used around the world for decades as a topical analgesic for treatment of arthritis pain. The analgesic property of DMSO combined with its ability to rapidly deliver drugs into tissues may be applicable to topical lidocaine. Some studies have determined that transdermal delivery of lidocaine is enhanced when DMSO is applied first.19 The pain suppression effect of lidocaine when dissolved in a 0.1% DMSO solution was markedly potentiated in another study.

A most intriguing investigation involved topical anesthesia in patients with vascular malformations who underwent typically painful pulsed dye laser treatments. Mallory et al21 mixed a 25% lidocaine base in 70% DMSO for topical application prior to laser treatments. Although this mixture did not produce total anesthesia, it was sufficient to allow patients to complete treatment with minimal discomfort rather than return several times for additional laser therapy. An in vitro permeation experiment found that lidocaine plus DMSO achieved significantly greater permeation of skin than did acid mantle cream or EMLA (AstraZeneca, Waltham, MA). Furthermore, no patient experienced stinging or itching at the lidocaine/DMSO application site, though there was transient mild erythema.

To avoid toxicity, limits to amounts of topical lidocaine need to be established, but the preparation used by Mallory et al included no more than 6 drops of 25% lidocaine, which is far less than the amount of drug delivered by injection.

If, with the addition of DMSO, topical lidocaine could be delivered into the skin more quickly, or if lower doses of lidocaine could be used, patients would greatly benefit. For example, patients would not have to wait as long before receiving painful injections, including tissue fillers, and suturing could be completed more quickly, and without lidocaine injection. This would be especially helpful for treating children. DMSO can carry nonionized molecules through skin if their molecular weight is less than 3000.

The molecular weight of lidocaine is 234.

Skin care applications

Using various dyes as visual tracers, followed by biopsies, a study of DMSO penetration into human skin demonstrated that the stratum corneum was completely stained.22 Thus, DMSO penetrated rapidly and deeply into the horny layer. This suggests that DMSO may increase the penetration of some facial peel chemicals down to the stratum corneum.

Antioxidants, such as vitamin C, are important components of good skin care. DMSO is perhaps the most powerful free radical scavenger—at least against hydroxyl—and a well tested carrier of other substances. Therefore, DMSO may have a role in skin rejuvenation. DMSO also inhibits bacteria growth,23 including Staphylococcus aureus, so it may be of benefit in treating acne.

An unfortunate side effect of DMSO used in any form (intravenous, injected, or topical) is that it causes a garlic-like breath odor that is not only unpleasant but also poses an "alert" that makes it difficult to conduct DMSO blinded clinical trials.13 Also, skin care products that caused a garlic-like breath odor would be a challenge to market.

DMSO is metabolized in humans by oxidation into dimethyl sulfone (MSM), or by reduction into dimethyl sulfide (DMS), both of which are excreted in urine and feces. DMS is eliminated through the breath and skin and is the metabolite responsible for the garlic odor of DMSO. Newer forms of DMSO, such as MSM, which is also known as DMSO2, are available that do not produce this odor, but they lack scientific testing. Dr. Stanley Jacob, considered the father of DMSO research, markets MSM and oral DMSO on his Web site (www.jacoblab.com) as a nutritional sulfur supplement ingested in liquid or crystal form. MSM or DMSO2 is probably also available in health food stores. Other Web sites sell MSM in capsule or powder form. These products apparently can be added to liquids for ingestion or mixed with distilled or deionized water or lotion for topical application. We do not know how the actions of these available MSM products compare with DMSO, but these products deserve further investigation

if they do eliminate the garlic odor.

DMSO and Free Radicals

DMSO is a small polar molecule (78 m.w.) with

sulfur in the center, 2 methyl groups, and an

oxygen atom at the apices. The oxygen atoms

carry a nonbinding electron pair.9 Its structure

makes DMSO soluble in aqueous and organic

media, and DMSO has become one of the most

common solvents for the in vivo administration

of water-insoluble substances.24 In fact, it is the only solvent that can effectively dissolve some hydrophobic drugs.

Reduces inflammatory activity of rheumatoid arthritis24 and ulcerative colitis26

Improves survival in patients with colon cancer27

Decreases collagen production in skin of scleroderma patients.

Reverses extravasation injury caused by chest-wall induration of chemotherapy.

Produces electromyographic evidence of muscle relaxation 1 hour after topical application.

Reduces experimental myocardial fiber necrosis and blocks calcium-induced degeneration of myocardial cells.

Reduces incidence of adhesions following serosal abrasions in the terminal ileum of rats.

Produces significant improvement in lower extremity function of patients with complex regional pain syndrome type I.

Reduces impairment of patients with reflex sympathetic dystrophy,

Treats adjuvant-induced polyarthritis of rats and significantly inhibits associated contact dermatitis, allergic eczema, and skin calcification

Reverses abnormal processing of LDL cholesterol in mutant Niemann-Pick disease fibroblasts

Reduces accumulation of cholesterol in vascular and extravascular tissues in rabbits

Inhibits growth of or inactivates bacteria, fungi, and viruses in vitro, and reduces drug resistance of some bacterial species.

Reduces inflammatory activity of rheumatoid arthritis and ulcerative colitis

Improves survival in patients with colon cancer

Decreases collagen production in skin of scleroderma patients.

Reverses extravasation injury caused by chest-wall induration of chemotherapy

Produces electromyographic evidence of muscle relaxation 1 hour after topical application

Reduces experimental myocardial fiber necrosis and blocks calcium-induced degeneration of myocardial cells

Reduces incidence of adhesions following serosal abrasions in the terminal ileum of rats

Produces significant improvement in lower extremity function of patients with complex regional pain syndrome type I

Reduces impairment of patients with reflex sympathetic dystrophy

Treats adjuvant-induced polyarthritis of rats and significantly inhibits associated contact dermatitis, allergic eczema, and skin calcification

Reverses abnormal processing of LDL cholesterol in mutant Niemann-Pick disease fibroblasts

Reduces accumulation of cholesterol in vascular and extravascular tissues in rabbits

Inhibits growth of or inactivates bacteria, fungi, and viruses in vitro, and reduces drug resistance of some bacterial species

Table 1Partial list of DMSO applications

Reduces inflammatory activity of rheumatoid arthritis and ulcerative colitis

Improves survival in patients with colon cancer

Decreases collagen production in skin of scleroderma patients

Reverses extravasation injury caused by chest-wall induration of chemotherapy

Produces electromyographic evidence of muscle relaxation 1 hour after topical application

Reduces experimental myocardial fiber necrosis and blocks calcium-induced degeneration of myocardial cells

Reduces incidence of adhesions following serosal abrasions in the terminal ileum of rats

Produces significant improvement in lower extremity function of patients with complex regional pain syndrome type I

Reduces impairment of patients with reflex sympathetic dystrophy

Treats adjuvant-induced polyarthritis of rats and significantly inhibits associated contact dermatitis, allergic eczema, and skin calcification

Reverses abnormal processing of LDL cholesterol in mutant Niemann-Pick disease fibroblasts

Reduces accumulation of cholesterol in vascular and extravascular tissues in rabbits

Inhibits growth of or inactivates bacteria, fungi, and viruses in vitro, and reduces drug resistance of some bacterial species

Reduces inflammatory activity of rheumatoid arthritis and ulcerative colitis

Improves survival in patients with colon cancer

Decreases collagen production in skin of scleroderma patients

Reverses extravasation injury caused by chest-wall induration of chemotherapy

Produces electromyographic evidence of muscle relaxation 1 hour after topical application

Reduces experimental myocardial fiber necrosis and blocks calcium-induced degeneration of myocardial cells

Reduces incidence of adhesions following serosal abrasions in the terminal ileum of rats

Produces significant improvement in lower extremity function of patients with complex regional pain syndrome type I

Reduces impairment of patients with reflex sympathetic dystrophy

Treats adjuvant-induced polyarthritis of rats and significantly inhibits associated contact dermatitis, allergic eczema, and skin calcification

Reverses abnormal processing of LDL cholesterol in mutant Niemann-Pick disease fibroblasts

Reduces accumulation of cholesterol in vascular and extravascular tissues in rabbits

Inhibits growth of or inactivates bacteria, fungi, and viruses in vitro, and reduces drug resistance of some bacterial species

Because of its small size and structure, DMSO molecules readily cross the membranes of skin, cells, and organelles.9 Furthermore, DMSO molecules can associate with a wide range of constituents, including water, proteins, carbohydrates, nucleic acid, and ionic substances. Radioactive tracer studies of DMSO absorption in humans found that 5 minutes after cutaneous application, DMSO is detectable in the blood; after 1 hour, it is detectable in the bones.

The free electron pairs of its oxygen atoms allow DMSO molecules to transfer electrons and accept hydrogen bonds. This structural characteristic makes DMSO a potent scavenger of free radicals, particularly hydroxyl (OH•), which is the most reactive free radical in biological systems. DMSO is such an effective scavenger because it is specific for OH• and can reach the sites of OH• generation, down to the mitochondrial level.

It is widely believed that the production of oxygen-derived free radicals is a major cause of ischemia and reperfusion injuries. The free radical scavenging ability of DMSO molecules also may figure prominently in the anti-inflammatory properties attributed to DMSO. The Table is a partial list of some medical applications of DMSO that have been published in peer-reviewed journals. A more complete list can be found in the articles by Santos et al24 and Jacob and Herschler.

DMSO and the FDA

The US Food and Drug Administration (FDA) halted all human studies of DMSO in 1965 when a woman in Ireland died of an allergic reaction after taking DMSO and several other drugs; however, her cause of death was never precisely determined. Also in 1965, pharmaceutical companies noted a refractive index change in the lenses of dogs, rabbits, and pigs treated with

DMSO at doses 50 to 100 times higher than typical doses used in humans. The lenses were not opaque, and no microscopic or chemical differences were detected. The lens problem was not observed in any humans or other primates who at that time were experimentally treated with DMSO in the United States or elsewhere. However, since pretreatment eye examinations had not been performed in patients receiving DMSO, the absence of lens changes could not be confirmed. The lens trouble in lower mammals was sufficient evidence for the FDA to conclude that DMSO was highly toxic, and almost all United States-based research was stopped. Since 1965 the FDA has permitted very little work with DMSO.

However, the FDA has approved DMSO as a preservative for transplant organs and for symptomatic relief of interstitial cystitis through intravesical instillation. DMSO is also approved as a component of pharmaceuticals, and its properties as a drug "carrier" are well known. Molecular weight, shape, and electrochemistry determine which drugs DMSO can effectively carry through cell membranes. In addition to these human uses, the FDA has approved topically applied DMSO for the treatment of musculoskeletal disorders in horses and dogs, and it is widely used in horse racing stables as a pain-relieving liniment.

In 1978 the FDA approved the use of DMSO alone for treatment of interstitial cystitis and other inflammatory conditions of the genitourinary tract, such as radiation cystitis and chronic prostatitis. Typically, RIMSO-50, a 50% solution of DMSO (Edwards Lifesciences, Irvine,

CA), is slowly instilled into the bladder with treatments repeated as frequently as needed to reduce symptoms. In one study, objective endoscopic improvement was seen in 85% of patients and 60% had an increase in bladder capacity.38 Because it lacks side effects, is inexpensive, and can be used in an office setting, intravesical DMSO is a treatment that may eliminate the need for surgery in many patients. It is believed that the anti-inflammatory and muscle relaxant properties of DMSO are responsible for the improvement in patients with interstitital cystitis.

A premarket approval application is currently before the FDA for the Onyx LES Liquid Embolic System (Micro Therapeutics, Inc., Irvine, CA), a device that incorporates DMSO for embolization of arteriovenous malformations in the brain. In this device, a mixture of ethylene vinyl alcohol copolymer and DMSO is delivered through a micro catheter to the target lesion and released to embolize the arteriovenous malformation. This Onyx system is currently used in Europe for intracranial aneurysms that cannot be treated with surgery or have not responded to other occlusion attempts.39 In this context, the FDA may be willing to approve the use of DMSO in a potentially life-saving device that requires minimal patient exposure.

DMSO and Toxicity

To address the FDA concern about lens changes in mammals and possible DMSO toxicity, a human study was undertaken in 1967-68. DMSO was administered to volunteers from a prison population in California who were involved in either a short-term (14 day) or long-term (90 day) study organized by Brobyn.40 A battery of tests were conducted before, during, and after the study start and stop points, including complete weekly physicals, ophthalmologic examinations, bone marrow studies, cerebrospinal fluid analysis, neurological exams (including electroencephalograms), pulmonary function studies, and electrocardiograph exams, as well as regular urine and blood analysis (including the full range of blood chemistries). The purpose of the tests was to look for hepatic, renal, or hematologic changes. The same examinations and testing regimen were administered to untreated controls at the same time intervals. In the experimental group, an 80% solution of DMSO gel was topically applied at 1 g/kg daily to 65 subjects for 14 days and to another 40 subjects for 90 days.

Data analysis revealed no significant differences among those receiving DMSO or the controls on any variable, with one exception: a small percentage of treated subjects had a slightly elevated peripheral eosinophil count. This eosinophilia was believed to result from the cutaneous histamine-releasing effect of DMSO. As expected, skin irritation (wheal and erythema with drying and scaling) was a common reaction to DMSO, but all reacting skin returned to normal within 3 weeks after treatment. No ocular or lens abnormalities occurred in the treated subjects.

Other investigations of lens abnormalities found no changes among patients with scleroderma treated with topical DMSO for 3 to 12 months.41,42 Nor did these studies find any other signs of possible systemic toxicity. The same was true in an investigation of rhesus monkeys given daily intravenous doses of 3 g/kg 40% DMSO for 9 consecutive days. The animals were examined during the following 4 months for changes in their eyes, blood chemistry, hematology, urine, and neurological and cardiovascular systems.43 After 4 months, the monkeys were sacrificed and received gross and microscopic pathological examinations. There were no significant differences between the monkeys that received DMSO compared with those that received intravenous saline.

Experiments have been performed to examine the toxicity and teratogenicity of various solvents used in medicine and pharmacology. In a study of frogs, DMSO was found to be the least toxic and least teratogenic solvent tested; formamide was the most toxic, and ethanol was the most teratogenic.44 Experiments exploring toxicity in mice have tested DMSO, polyethylene glycol 400 (PEG 400), dimethylformamide (DMF), absolute ethanol (EtOH), and benzyl alcohol (BeOH).45 There were no major differences in acute toxicity of the solvents in 3 mouse strains, although DMSO was less toxic in 1 strain, and BeOH and EtOH were less toxic in the other 2 strains.

The Brobyn prison study demonstrated that even though topical DMSO does not seem to be toxic when given at doses 3 to 30 times the typical human dose for up to 3 months, it is not without side effects. In addition to skin irritation, daily high-dose dermal application produced sedation and occasional insomnia or nausea in a small number of subjects. Even fewer men in the treated group reported dizziness or diarrhea.40 Intravenous administration of DMSO is more likely to produce adverse reactions, though they are uncommon; examples include red cell lysis with DMSO concentrations above 40%,46 and hypernatremia with fluid overload when DMSO concentrations were 10% or less.47 Allergic reactions are rarely reported.24

DMSO and Tissue Perfusion

Several different mechanisms may explain how DMSO counteracts ischemia after trauma. It is believed that DMSO protects the integrity of cell membranes during injury,48 especially defending against attack by hydroxyl radicals, which are generated at a high level after ischemic injury. This ability to preserve cell membranes may partially explain how DMSO improves cerebral and spinal cord blood flow

after injury.49 In experimental cerebral ischemia,
DMSO prevents or breaks up platelet
aggregation,50 which may either promote
ischemia or extend it. DMSO also has been found
to prevent thrombus formation in vivo.

One of the more intriguing characteristics of
DMSO is its potential to increase perfusion in
injured tissues. Investigators have been studying
this application of DMSO in cerebral ischemia
since the 1970s.51–54 To examine DMSO in a
clinical setting, 20 patients in Turkey with severe
closed head injuries were given intravenous

DMSO.55,56 In both studies (10 patients per study) DMSO rapidly reduced intracranial pressure, increased cerebral perfusion pressure and blood flow, and improved outcomes so that most patients had no residual deficits.

Experimental studies of animals have found that, in addition to the brain and spinal cord, DMSO reduces the damage caused by ischemia in other organs. Intravenous DMSO was very effective in reversing acute ischemic renal failure in rats.57 DMSO increased myocardial perfusion in dogs58 and rats59 and has effectively improved liver perfusion after microvascular injury in rats, probably by reducing leukocyte adhesion to the sinusoidal wall.60

DMSO on the World Wide Web

Because DMSO is an organic solvent with multiple applications in industry and medicine, it is readily available throughout the United States. As news of its potential medical applications has spread through lay publications, DMSO has gained popularity in the unregulated world of homeopathic remedies and health and nutrition outlets. It can be purchased in some health food stores and through hundreds (if not thousands) of Web sites at a concentration of 70% or 90% for less than $10.00 for an 8-ounce bottle. Gels and creams are also available. Web sites typically contain a disclaimer, such as this one from www.smartbomb.com: "Ninety-nine % pure DMSO. This product is intended for use as a solvent only. The choice of the process used in the various applications is the sole responsibility of the user."

Some applications of DMSO touted on the Web are so absurd that they are comical. DMSO and MSM capsules allegedly treat or prevent allergies and asthma, back pain, carpal tunnel syndrome, constipation, diarrhea, depression, diabetes, emphysema, heartburn, hypertension, infection, leg cramps, migraines, parasites, and sinusitis. Further, claims are made that it reduces wrinkles, grows hair in balding areas, and stimulates DNA repair. Unfortunately, these kinds of claims can only confuse the actual and valuable applications of DMSO in medicine.

Finally, the FDA status of DMSO is somewhat reminiscent of the history of silicone gel–filled breast implants. DMSO got a reputation for toxicity in 1965 that has not been overcome, even though studies have determined that lens changes do not occur in humans or other primates treated with DMSO. The lack of approved uses for DMSO may have tragic consequences. Injections of DMSO into the spinal cord soon after injury have shown great promise for restoring function. Furthermore, the use of DMSO for treating closed head injuries is not an option in the United States, and no FDA-approved clinical trials are currently underway.

At the same time, we find no instances of the FDA warning physicians not to use DMSO. Furthermore, since people have the choice of self-medicating with DMSO, it is difficult to imagine a pharmaceutical company willing to do the work required to determine what the actual value of DMSO might be. Good experimental and anecdotal evidence indicates that DMSO increases tissue perfusion and may effectively treat or prevent ischemia in flaps. The application of DMSO cannot salvage every

compromised flap, but we have witnessed its

benefits when used on flaps that show signs of

ischemia.

Other Incredible Benefits of DMSO

DMSO for Cancer

One 2012 study of DMSO demonstrated that it may be an important stimulator of the tumor suppressor protein HLJ1 through AP-1 activation in highly invasive lung adenocarcinoma cells. Previous studies had demonstrated that using DMSO could modulate AP-1 activity and lead to cell cycle arrest at the G1 phase. While nothing is conclusive (yet), according to this study, targeted induction of the HLJ1 represents a promising approach for cancer therapy. This means that DMSO could serve as a potential lead compound as anticancer drugs are developed in the future.

Early research has also suggested that injecting DMSO intravenously along with sodium bicarbonate can help alleviate cancer-related pain.

DMSO for Pain

DMSO is known to address a variety of types of pain. Strains and sprains are one type of pain that DMSO can address. When used topically, DMSO can eliminate the pain of these types of injuries. DMSO will pass through the skin's oily membranes and reduce swelling and inflammation in the area.

DMSO can also be effective for pain related to bruises, burns, scars, and keloids. A concentration of 50 to 80 percent DMSO put on two to three times per day can flatten a raised scar and eliminate burns and bruising.

DMSO for Arthritis

Early research has suggested that applying DMSO topically may help decrease the symptoms of both types of arthritis – osteoarthritis (OA) and rheumatoid (RA). This is likely due to DMSO's ability to penetrate tissues.

DMSO for Extravasations

Using DMSO has been shown to help with drug extravasation injury. Extravasation refers to the escape of a drug into the extravascular space (soft tissue), either by leakage from a vessel or by direct infiltration. Research suggests this is beneficial to chemotherapy patients as chemotherapy drugs can leave into surrounding tissues (extravasate), and the effects can be highly damaging to the body. For affected patients, DMSO application can significantly improve the tissue injury that occurs from extravasation.

DMSO for Complex Regional Pain Syndrome

Complex regional pain syndrome (CRPS) is a chronic pain condition that often effects one limb after an injury. It is believed to be caused by damage or malfunction to the peripheral and central nervous systems. Research suggests that applying a 50 percent DMSO cream to the skin improves pain in people with CRPS.

DMSO for Atherosclerosis

Atherosclerosis is a disease in which plaque builds up inside your arteries. As a result, oxygen-rich blood flow is limited to both your organs and other parts of your body. Typical treatments involve lifestyle challenges like a healthy diet and exercise. In laboratory testing, DMSO has demonstrated its ability to delay the development of narrowing arteries induced by dietary cholesterol. It also suppresses the accumulation of cholesterol in tissues, despite severely elevated levels.

DMSO for Interstitial Cystitis

Interstitial cystitis is a chronic condition causing pressure, bladder pain, and sometimes pelvic pain. The condition is part of a spectrum of diseases known as painful bladder syndrome. Unfortunately, chronic pain often makes it difficult to deal with. Fortunately, instilling DMSO – an in-office procedure in which medication is injected into the bladder through a urinary catheter – is an FDA-approved pain-relieving treatment.

DMSO for Shingles

Shingles is a viral infection that causes a painful rash. It is caused by varicella-zoster, which is the same virus that causes chickenpox. Anyone who's had chickenpox may develop shingles, and because risk increases with age (most people are older than 50 when they get it), it is often considered the adult version of the chickenpox.

All that said, shingles is painful, and DMSO has been found to be helpful in a variety of ways. If you apply DMSO to the skin along with a drug called idoxuridine, your lesions and swelling associated with shingles may lessen. Additionally, research indicates that applying this same combination to the skin can also help to reduce pain.

DMSO for Scleroderma

Scleroderma is a chronic connective tissue disease in which the skin hardens. Because DMSO penetrates the skin, doctors initially tested the effects of DMSO on scleroderma to see what would happen. DMSO was found to have anti-inflammatory effects while continuing to increase blood supply to the skin.

DMSO for High Blood Pressure

High blood pressure is a primary or contributing cause of death in 2017 for almost half a million people in the United States. When using DMSO intravenously, it can be used to lower abnormally high blood pressure.

DMSO Benefits even help with spinal cord injuries

People who sustain head or spinal cord injuries have seen results when their doctors give them an intravenous dose of DMSO shortly after their injury. According to research, the sooner this is given the more likely the person is to recover with no residual side effects such as paralysis.

Heart patients who have had a heart attack or struggle with severe angina attacks have found great relief when given DMSO by IV. Since the DMSO-dissolves blood clots and works to clear arteries, patients are given a better prognosis.

Alzheimer and Parkinson's patients have found relief from trembling when they are given DMSO. It crosses the blood barrier to the brain and works as dopamine to help reduce trembling and it can help regenerate portions of the brain where damage has occurred and caused damage. For those who suffer easily from viruses, the DMSO works in conjunction with antibiotics to dissolve the proteins surrounding the viruses and render them inert. People will recover more quickly.

Dentists who apply it on their patient's sore gums and teeth report that their patients are recovering more quickly and report fewer gum infections. Anyone who has suffered from a painful bout of gout, corns or calluses on their feet will appreciate the fact that it helps reduce painful foot conditions and works to heal the injured area. DMSO has established itself as a more effective and safer choice than synthetic drugs and clearly shows the many DMSO Benefits that patients are reporting.

DMSO Frequently Asked Questions

Is DMSO toxic to humans?

DMSO is no more toxic to humans than any other supplement as long as it is used properly. We recommend that you always start low and slow to see how you react to DMSO.

 Is DMSO FDA Approved?

The FDA has approved DMSO as a prescription medication for treating symptoms of painful bladder syndrome. It's also used under medical supervision to treat several other conditions, including shingles. The bottles sold over the counter are labeled not for human use.

Is DMSO Safe?

Yes, it is considered generally safe. However, any product can be used incorrectly. You should always consult with your Holistic Health Practitioner to go over your particular situation. You should also purchase DMSO from a reputable provider to ensure you are getting pharmaceutical-grade DMSO.

Is there any situation that I should not use DMSO?

You should not use DMSO if you have any type of medical implant, such as breast implants, or any other medical device without medical supervision.

Can I use DMSO on my pets?

Yes. DMSO has been used on pets for years.

Does DMSO cure some cancers?

www.ingramcontent.com/pod-product-compliance
Lightning Source LLC
Chambersburg PA
CBHW061055250726
48653CB00001B/417